Learn the AB... your Awareness, Body Confidence & Courage

PERSONAL

SAFETY TIPS

EVERY WOMAN

SHOULD KNOW

A POCKET GUIDE

LILA REYNA

www.LilaReyna.com

Published by: BookLight Publishing

ISBN (print): 978-1-7337407-2-2
ISBN (e-book): 978-1-7337407-3-9

Printed in the United States of America

Originally published in 2011 under the title *Your Life in Your Hands*. Updated to better complement my workshops and trainings.

Contents

Awareness is prevention.
Prevention is your #1 defense.

Introduction

Developing an effective self-defense strategy means more than preparing yourself with self-defense devices or learning fighting techniques. First and foremost, enhancing your personal safety includes cultivating a mentality of awareness and street smarts that can be relied upon in the heat of a real-life situation.

Having an awareness of your environment and the people within it—and understanding *your* actions and reactions—are important aspects of staying safe in a world where crime and violence are a reality.

- According to The National Women's Study, 683,000 forcible rapes occur every year in the United States, which equals 56,916 per month; 1,871 per day; 78 per hour; and 1.3 per minute.[1]

- One in 12 women will be stalked in their lifetime.[2]

- One in 5 women will be raped in their lifetime.[3]

- In the United States, one woman is beaten by her husband or partner every 15 seconds,[4] which makes domestic violence the leading cause of injury to women between the ages of 15 and 44.[5]

While these figures are shocking and it is good to be aware of them, we are not here to focus on statistics—learning how *not* to become a statistic is more important. The following pages detail various modes of defense that are available to you. Keep in mind that no one can guarantee a specific tactic will work for you all of the time or in every location. Take the time to consider and evaluate your options now, because if you are ever confronted, there will be little or no time to think about those options during the attack.

Even though violence touches all of us, and we all have ways to contribute to preventing violence, you may turn a blind eye to it because the reality can be disheartening or bring up fears. You may even ask yourself, "Why learn about violence and safety when we have police officers to protect the streets and trained government officials to ensure our safety?" But the truth is this: your safety is up to you, and no one is immune to violence.

It is not the job of the police, the government, your spouse, boss, or a security company. Your safety is your responsibility.

The foundation of my Action Awareness Training A-B-C Defense program is practicing **A**wareness, **B**ody Confidence, and **C**ourage. This preventative defense is based on knowledge and intuition, not muscle. The A-B-C approach enables a woman to connect with her individual strength, power, and belief in herself, which are the essential components of lifelong survival skills.

Personal Safety Tips Every Woman Should Know is a powerful resource that can help you protect yourself and your loved ones. It was written to be a fast and informative read for all women who want to enhance their awareness and take control of their own personal safety.

Part One: The A-B-C Approach to Safety

Chapter One
Engaging the Mind: Awareness

We don't know how long she was lying face-down in the alley with her hands bound together and a rag stuffed into her mouth, but we do know that three men gang-raped Sara while she lay half-conscious and unable to defend herself.

Sara was walking her dog in a nearby neighborhood at three in the afternoon. She had the fleeting thought to cross the street when the three men eyeing her from the sidewalk ahead made her feel uncomfortable, but she chose to walk on. As she walked by the men, Sara laughed to herself, feeling silly that she had felt at all uneasy.

Then, suddenly, she was struck on the back of the head and thrown into a small alleyway between two houses. She lost consciousness, only to wake up to an emergency medical personnel untying what was binding her wrists together above her head. It was her dog's leash.

When someone is trying to harm you, you won't have time to carefully work out what to do, but thinking ahead about possible scenarios and what-ifs and learning safety tips can help you be prepared. Thinking about safety issues also promotes prevention. Although there are no absolutes and nothing works every time, there are preventative measures we can learn—and take—that are based on awareness and knowledge.

Acknowledging that crime does happen and that it can happen to you is the first step to protecting yourself. Crime can happen to *anyone*. We install fire alarms to protect ourselves and our possessions, check references before hiring babysitters, and install burglar alarms in our homes, so why do we not all take self-defense classes? Because no one thinks it can happen to them. But the reality is that no one is immune to the threat of violence. Without warning, a situation can turn from safe to sorry, turning you not only into a victim, but into the top news story of the day.

Most people who are victimized never imagined that crime could or would happen to them. We think, "It always happens to the other person, not me!" Simply acknowledging that crime happens and that it could happen to you at any given moment is the first step in owning your personal safety.

Just as anyone can be a victim, anyone can be an assailant. Assailants do not have an easy-to-read banner across their foreheads that reads "criminal." It's important to understand that they can look and dress like any of us. For example, an assailant can look like the suit-and-tie serial killer of the 1960s, Ted Bundy, who charmed, raped, and killed his victims and then returned to the crime sites days later to engage in sex with the corpses. They can look like Paul Bernardo and Karla Homolka, a young couple who teamed up and raped and murdered three young women, including Karla's own younger sister. They can look like the Milwaukee cannibal Jeffery Dahmer, who from 1978 to 1991 raped, strangled, and then severed and ate his victims so that he could always feel close to them. They may look like college student Dzhokhar Tsarnaev, the Boston marathon bomber, or Ian David Long, who opened fire in a music bar in Thousand Oaks, California, in 2018, killing twelve innocent people.

In short, an assailant can look, dress, and act like anyone— like you or like me. They can be male or female and work individually or in teams.

A common way you may be approached is by a woman who may ask you a question, such as directions to a store. For the most part, women are more comfortable being approached by other women, so we may automatically let our guard down when a woman approaches us compared to when a man approaches us. And we are conditioned to answer questions, so immediately our brain switches to answer mode. When that happens, your awareness often switches focus, too. As you focus on the woman and your response, it's easy to miss her partner in crime run up from behind, grab your purse, and then run off with it. Worse yet, the accomplice may grab you in a chokehold and drag you into their vehicle.

Throughout this book, you will learn tips and tools that you can pair with your intuition to enhance your awareness and hone your personal safety tactics.

The Crime Triangle

The crime triangle helps us understand how crime happens. By understanding the process, you can greatly reduce your chances of becoming a victim. From the predator's viewpoint, there are three components to making crime happen: *desire, target,* and *opportunity.* The good news is that you have control over two out of the three.

Any crime starts with desire, and that comes from the intent and motivation of the predator. Realistically, you have no control over this part, but you do have a say as soon as the desire turns into a physical search for a target and an opportunity. This is where you come in.

The target is *you.* The target is anyone who appears to be an easy victim. Even a predator doesn't want to put up a fight for what they want—instead, they look for easy pickings to reduce the chance of a struggle. An easy victim is someone who is unaware of her surroundings and appears to be easy to overpower. To reduce the chances of being targeted as an easy victim, always keep your eyes up and scan the area around you. Stand tall with your shoulders back and walk with energy and confidence.

The third aspect of any crime is opportunity. This, too, you have some control over, because you can pay attention to your environment. What kind of people are you hanging out with? Are you letting strangers or acquaintances ask too many questions and get in your personal space? Are you in a bad part of town or in a secluded area? Limiting opportunity is about paying attention to your environment and listening to your intuition, and then actively removing yourself from a situation if necessary.

Building Self-Awareness

In our society in general, most of us have become somewhat detached from trusting our inner "gut feelings." In place of intuition, we often rely on information that is dictated by the media, and other external sources that endorse the normalcy of a situation. We tend to trust government, experts, and technologies like personal safety apps, 911, and pepper spray over our own feelings and natural abilities. It's easy to invest our confidence in external sources without ever evaluating those sources; and besides, not being accountable for our own safety also makes it easy to place blame on others if there ever is an issue. But the *true* key to personal safety is being in tune with your intuition and building your self-awareness.

Self-awareness is when you become mindful of yourself, your experiences, your thoughts, your feelings, your intentions, and your actions. Perhaps the reason we pay so little attention to ourselves is that doing so interrupts the way we ordinarily engage with the world—we are often taught to focus on the external world while only remaining partially aware of our internal feelings. Cultivating self-awareness challenges us to go beyond those typical considerations and seek to identify what is fallacy and what is truth.

Over the years, we have invented incredible technologies and devices such as the internet, video games, and cell phones. We've also come up with countless ways to combine foods to satisfy our palates and drugs to calm our pain. The temptations that these external stimulations offer redirect our focus and awareness on an external object (which often becomes a distraction) rather than encouraging us to explore our feelings and gain a better understanding of the core issue at hand. Virtually all of our lives are spent in what I will call the "common consciousness." In our common consciousness, we regard ourselves as being passive receptors of an external and independently existing world. In this state, our attention is directed outward, toward the world with which we are engaged, and away from the self as an instrument of knowing and doing. In a way, we have lost some of our connection to the self; we have partially lost our ability to communicate with, accept, and especially *trust* our inner voice.

In our common consciousness, we live a life based on conditioned responses, and we react to our surrounding environments and situations rather than existing in a state of intention and awareness. In the unmindful state of our common consciousness, we find ourselves in circumstances which do not necessarily allow us to choose the outcome—often, we allow the outcome to choose *us*. This can be seen in many relationships, especially abusive partnerships. When someone is the victim of abuse, it can be hard for them to identify with the self because of the intense mixed emotions surrounding the situation. If we are too caught up in living from a place of emotional reaction, rather than active awareness, that lack of awareness can create huge blind spots and hinder our ability to anticipate and perceive potentially dangerous situations.

In a way, we become transformed by society so that we can fit in the way that people *expect* us to fit in. The good news is that each of us can change our mindset—we can go from being stuck in the common consciousness to embracing our self-awareness. Making that transition takes patience, though, and it takes believing that you are worth it.

Activating Awareness

The *Stop, Look, and Listen* method[6] is a three-step approach that encourages the mind to engage in the moment. This is the precursor to becoming self-aware. Taking the time to be cognizant of your actions and reactions will redirect in-the-moment conditioned responses into conscious awareness. Taking the time to stop, look, and listen activates awareness. Remember, awareness is our number-one defense. Engage the mind by using *Stop, Look, and Listen.*

1. **STOP** and APPRECIATE

Before we can look and listen, first we must STOP. Take time out and "smell the roses." The world can be a quiet place, and you can take a moment to be quiet, too. No cars, no traffic, no screaming children, no challenging teenagers, no stress, no deadlines to meet...all right, realistically, life is probably never going to be *that* quiet, but the important point is that even amongst all the little to-do lists and major stresses we all have (both positive and negative), we can take time to slow down and appreciate life's details. Appreciating our environment and our external accommodations as well as appreciating our inner strengths (and our weaknesses, too) is the first step toward gaining awareness.

"Smell the roses" isn't just an old saying from the past—it's still a valuable skill! Awareness begins with the act of appreciating the simple pleasures in life. Simplicity has a way of centering the self, grounding the self, and getting the self away from all of the distracting technologies in our lives. Simplicity reminds us that we are all connected. Most importantly, simplicity reminds us of the value of connecting with ourselves.

Stop taking yourself so seriously and have some fun! Get out and enjoy life. Have a good laugh! Yes, it's easier said than done. Especially for women—we naturally juggle many tasks at once while often stretching our attention beyond the task at hand. That ability comes in handy when you're on an important business call and your two-year-old suddenly falls and bumps his head just as the oven timer reminds you it's time to pull out tonight's dinner, or when you're in the car and the cell phone rings and your best friend decides to download her dramatic day as you're desperately trying to apply lipstick while driving to meet your date.

But too much multitasking and taking your life too seriously can also squeeze out your self-awareness, thus creating a victim in the works. You become a victim to the chatter of the common consciousness that can dull even the sharpest of minds. If you neglect to take the time to stop and acknowledge what your body or mind is, or is not, reacting to, then you wind up stuck in a blinded reality. And no one wants to be blindsided.

There are as many ways to achieve this first step of awareness as there are different people in the world, so you'll have to figure out what works best for you. But here are a few simple starter suggestions to help you stop, slow down, and appreciate life:

- Get up an extra 45 minutes before everyone else in the house does so that you can enjoy a cup of coffee with no distractions. This time alone in the morning can get the entire day off to a good start and help create a more balanced you.

- Set aside a minimum of 20 minutes of your day to go on a walk, practice yoga, or engage in some form of exercise. This gets the blood pumping and induces a natural high.

- Take 10 minutes before bed or early in the morning to breathe deeply, pray, or meditate. Concentrating on the breath can quiet the mind and relax the body.

- Make time to read your favorite book or soak up some sun.

- Stop putting everyone else before yourself—instead, put yourself at the top of your "to-do" list. This is not a selfish act, but a necessary one that will allow you to recharge yourself and remain in balance. Take care of you!

Setting aside a few minutes of pleasure for yourself can go a long way. Everyone from family members to friends to colleagues will benefit from a happy and well-adjusted woman. And if you find yourself in a dangerous situation, it's easier to assess and react to the situation if you have a calm and centered mind.

If you're walking down the street and the hair on the back of your neck rises or a creepy and uncomfortable feeling overcomes you, this is when the "stop" part of *Stop, Look, and Listen* comes into play. Stop whatever it is you are doing or thinking. Center yourself so that the situation at hand can be looked at from a grounded and aware perspective, one that will improve the possibility of the situation having a safe outcome.

To "stop" can be used throughout your daily routine or it can be applied within a split second, depending on the intensity or danger of your circumstances. Once you slow down and stop, the next step is to look.

2. **LOOK** and ACKNOWLEDGE

LOOK means assessing a situation from as many viewpoints and perspectives as possible. Visually look around you. What kind of environment are you in? If you are in a building, where are the exits and how many are there? What kind of people are around you and what are they doing? Are they happy, solemn, in an argument, on the phone, or sitting on a bench? You don't always have to understand what they are doing—your job is simply to take note of what's happening around you. If you are on the street, notice the vehicles around you, the people passing by, and all other activities, even if nothing seems suspicious. Look in front of you, to the side, and behind you, first looking at what's closest to you and then looking as far as the eye can see.

To increase your ability to look for and observe potentially threatening situations, also look within and practice self-awareness. Being aware of your inner self and knowing what makes you tick gives you an advantage and allows you to better see the good, the bad, and the ugly. The stronger your self-awareness is, the easier it is to perceive, navigate past, and avoid threatening situations. In the realm of self-awareness, to look means to acknowledge your feelings and to know your strengths and weaknesses.

Take a deeper look at yourself. If you are confronted with a real-life threatening situation, you don't want to have *two* strangers attacking you, so get to know yourself by answering the questions on the following page.

1. If a challenging situation arises, my first response is to handle it with: a) an emotional outburst, b) my intellect, or c) my intuition.

2. In general, how confident do I feel day-to-day on a 1–10 scale (with 10 being the highest rating)?

3. If an assailant approaches me, how confident am I that I can physically protect myself, on a 1–10 scale?

4. Am I typically a leader or a follower? Give an example.

5. What do I like about myself?

6. What would I like to change about myself?

7. What do I consider to be my main weakness?

8. What is my strongest attribute?

9. How aware am I of my surroundings, on a 1–10 scale?

10. If someone threatening approaches me, how confident am I that I can raise my voice and yell at them, on a 1–10 scale?

Grab a journal and take some time to write down your answers. If you're not happy with how you answered a question, what can you do to improve your response and feel better about it? For example, if you gave yourself a 3 for your ability to physically defend yourself, maybe it's time to invest in a self-defense workshop. If you have a difficult time using your voice, try taking singing lessons, acting lessons, debate workshops, or anything that involves speaking up.

Now, for an interesting twist, pass these same questions along to at least three other people who know you and ask them to answer them on your behalf. Their answers may surprise you and give insight about what you are truly projecting, not just what you *think* you are showing the world. Sometimes who we feel we are and how we actually project ourselves are complete opposites.

Then, after you've stopped and looked, it's time to listen.

3. **LISTEN** and TAKE ACTION

Your mind and body act together as a warning system that helps promote your safety and well-being. The more often you listen and observe, the more you will learn about your own behaviors and reactions as well as the behaviors and reactions of others. When you are able to stop, look, and then listen to your thoughts, moods, and behaviors, you naturally become more responsible for your actions. This in turn gives you an understanding of why and when others may react, thus preventing you from ending up in a dangerous situation to begin with.

One way to take action is to listen to your "natural navigator," which is your intuition or your gut instinct. Intuition is the ability to have a sense, vision, or feeling about someone or something. Intuition communicates with us through symbols, feelings, or simply a sense of knowing. It usually doesn't speak to us in clear language, at least not in the way you might expect to "hear" messages.

Intuition gives us the power to obtain knowledge that cannot otherwise be acquired by observation, reason, or experience. Because of this (and because they are often fleeting feelings), intuitive thoughts are often dismissed as simply being random or inconsequential. It can be quite frustrating when we are getting the message but not getting any logical reasoning along with it.

However, if you begin to follow through on your intuitive hunches, it's like you're taking test drives and honing your listening skills. The more we listen to our inner dialogue, the more natural it becomes to pay attention to it and to ourselves.

When we choose to ignore our gut instincts, we are limiting ourselves and our built-in natural navigator.

Intuition may manifest itself in different ways for different people. For some, it may come as "voices in the head," visions, or answers in dreams. It may be a feeling: a sense of knowing, feeling uncomfortable or scared, having butterflies in the stomach or pressure in the chest, or being peaceful, happy, and calm. It may manifest as aches and pains in the body or as tingling. You may see sudden colors or shadows. There is no right or wrong way to feel your intuition—it can be unique to each individual.

To polish your natural intuitive abilities, start small so that you will be able to identify the way your intuition works for you. (And remember, intuition can work in multiple ways.) Ask yourself what you feel in your heart. Do what you *feel*, not what you *think* is right. Everyone has the ability to receive natural intuition, but the tricky part is to listen, trust, and then follow through by taking action.

What stops us from listening to and trusting our intuition?

- The brain nerd: The logical mind wants proof and facts.

- Ms. Doubt: At first, it's common to wonder if it's really intuition or just a thought.

- Social conditioning: Most of us aren't raised with or encouraged to use our intuition.

- "Hear only what you want to hear" syndrome: Sometimes our intuition comes through loud and clear, but if we don't like what it's telling us, we disregard it.

- Self-sabotage: When our intuition pops up, the inner critic is quick to offer its sabotaging opinion.

> Self-sabotage can be subtle, but it is a form of self-victimization and can have a detrimental effect on how you live your life.

Think about it: not understanding why you do what you do or feel what you feel is like going through your life with a stranger's mind. How can you listen to your intuition and make healthy decisions and choices if you don't understand *why* you want what you want? Never knowing what the stranger inside of you is going to do next is a challenging and chaotic way to live. Get to know yourself and learn to trust your intuition by starting with the exercises below.

- Capture snapshots of the day through journal writing. Write down your responses and feelings. Journal about your inner dialogues and everything you notice within and outside of yourself.

- Note the patterns of your thoughts and reactions. Observe your behavior when you are under pressure. What do you do when someone pushes your buttons? How do you talk to yourself outwardly and inwardly? Do you go into a rage, or do you hide under the covers? Do you blame yourself or others? Listen to your reactions from an observer's point of view.

- When communicating with others, listen carefully. Listen with all of your senses and get a quick read on the situation. If someone's words don't match the emotion behind them, listen to your intuition. A quick assessment will allow you to feel the other person's energy, be aware of any subtle changes, and adjust accordingly. Ask yourself questions like, "Is this person potentially dangerous?," "Do they want something from me?," and "Are they sucking my energy?"

- With friends, practice accepting feedback without defending yourself. If you do this, you're more likely to hear what you need to hear, not just what you want to hear.
- Pay attention and listen to self-talk. What are you telling yourself? Communicate with your consciousness by asking questions—and then listen for answers.

Listen with your intuition and your logical mind. When you use these two essential parts of yourself in a balanced way, you'll have a well-rounded understanding of a given situation, and that understanding will create the awareness you need to succesfully maintain your personal safety.

Exercises to Engage the Mind

- **Test your awareness!** Did you notice that "successfully" was misspelled at the end of the previous sentence? Our mind often scans over what we think should be in front of us rather than observing the truth.

- **Test your intuition when you walk, ride, or pull up to a stoplight.** Practice predicting when the light will turn colors before it changes. Small games like this can increase your intuition.

- **Take the restaurant quiz.** When you go out to eat, observe every detail. Afterward, have a friend ask you questions like "What color was the rug?" or "What was the hostess wearing?" or "Who was sitting behind you?"

- **Get to know yourself.** Ask yourself, "What do I want in life? What motivates me? What makes me happy? What are my beliefs and values?"

- **Keep challenging your mind.** Learn something new—don't let your mind get bored! Play chess, decode a Rubik's cube, or learn a foreign language.

Chapter Two

Educating the Body: Body Confidence

What are we really communicating to the world? Body confidence develops through awareness of body language, knowledge of physical techniques, and being in tune with your body.

Body language is the silent talk that tells all. We gauge a person's body language to decipher their mood or demeanor in order to get a "feel" for them before they speak. If someone is angry, they don't have to aggressively shout, "Leave me alone—I'm angry!" The clenched jaw, white knuckles, or fists pounding on a table tells us that this person needs space to cool down. If someone is nervous, they don't have to whisper "I'm nervous" in our ear for us to understand that they're uneasy. They may pace back and forth or repetitively tap their fingers, or they may become quiet and reserved. Others may turn up the volume, cracking jokes and laughing loudly in an effort to try to hide their nervousness.

That said, the way we communicate is constantly changing in tandem with the rapid proliferation of technological devices, which is both good and bad. For example, instant messaging and texting are fast and fun ways to communicate, but they can also create unnecessary problems because of their lack of nuance. Words are simply a mix-up of letters, until we perceive more than just those letters and assign emotions to them. When we receive a text, we are unable to read the sender's body language or hear the spoken tone or inflection of their remark. This can lead to hasty, reckless, and sometimes regrettable reactions. Talking on the phone can help reduce misconstrued perceptions because we can at least hear the fluctuations of someone's voice—plus spoken communication can progress in ongoing, full sentences with back-and-forth dialogue, rather than in abbreviated, fast chit-chat.

Communicating healthy body language increases our personal safety by powerfully projecting a non-victim demeanor. A potential attacker is already in a weakened state, having a mindset that includes low self-esteem along with feelings of insecurity and not being in control. In order to get their desired power fix, they must succeed with their attack. That is why they look for someone who appears to be weaker than themselves. Easier targets are the ones who appear vulnerable.

Often, our body language expresses how we're feeling in the moment. If you look strong, alert, and healthy, you have a much better chance of being left alone. Effective body language conveys a relaxed sense of confidence—when you have control over your nonverbal language, you can communicate confidence without even having to say anything.

The suggestions below may seem inconsequential, but they can make an enormous difference when it comes to being a targeted victim or remaining safe.

Tips for Projecting Confidence

1. Stand or sit tall and proud.

2. Walk with intent and purpose.

3. Keep your eyes and head elevated at all times.

4. Uncross your arms and keep your hands out of your pockets so you can defend yourself if needed.

5. If you're feeling emotional, don't let it show until you're in the security of your own home.

6. Look at your surroundings (including around and behind you) to show you are aware.

7. Stop fidgeting – unintentional gestures are emotional reactions and are the result of the body's desire for comfort. Fidgeting is an anxious behavior and can make others around you uneasy.

8. Keep your shoulders back to help you look strong.

9. Swing your arms. This makes you look bigger and takes up more space in front of and behind you.

10. If you're walking with a group of people, remind them about the power of body language so that your group is strong and doesn't look like an easy target.

The Body Language of Others

Just as an assailant watches for vulnerable victim-mode body language, *you* can observe others for pre-attack body language. Doing so can help you avoid or de-escalate aggressive behavior. "Approximately 65% of communication consists of nonverbal behaviors. Of the remaining 35%, inflection, pitch, and loudness account for more than 25%, while less than 7% of communication has to do with what the person is verbally saying."[7]

Pre-Attack Warning Signs

1. Strange eye movements: Watch for darting eyes, glistening eyes (indicating distress), contracting pupils (indicating agitation), a tendency to break eye contact, a thousand-yard stare (they look right through you), and jerky eye movement (could be experiencing hallucinations).

2. Quickening of breath.

3. Darkening of the face.

4. Opening and closing hands.

5. Shaking, twitching, or rocking of the body.

6. Excessive talking or sudden silence.

7. Bulging veins or heavy sweating.

8. Finger-tapping or toe-tapping.

9. Suddenly rising from a sitting position.

10. Target glancing: This could mean that they are checking to see if you are armed or may be thinking about where to strike you.

If you notice one or more pre-attack indicators, create some distance, disengage, and move to a safe area. If you're not able to relocate, then your next line of defense—along with strengthening your body language—is using your voice. In a self-defense scenario, fighting is a last-resort tactic and should only be used after all other tactics have failed or you have reason to believe that all other tactics *will* fail. Just using your voice and sternly yelling, "Stop!" or "Stay back!" or "Don't mess with me!" is enough to show an attacker that you're not an easy victim. They will often have second thoughts about attacking an assertive woman.

How to De-Escalate a Situation

De-escalating a situation means speaking or acting in a way that can prevent things from getting worse. Effective de-escalation techniques feel odd because we are intuitively driven into fight-or-flight mode when scared. With de-escalation, however, we can neither fight nor flee—we must appear calm and centered even when terrified. That is why it's a good idea to practice these techniques beforehand so that they can become second nature. While de-escalating another person, you want to be in a non-threatening, non-challenging, self-protecting position.

Nonverbal De-Escalation Techniques

1. Maintain calm eye contact. An intense stare may be interpreted as aggressive which may add fuel to the fire. On the other hand, a loss of eye contact may be interpreted as an expression of fear or rejection or a lack of interest.

2. Maintain a relaxed and upright posture. Avoid aggressive stances.

3. Maintain a neutral facial expression. A calm, attentive expression reduces hostility.

4. Minimize body movements like shifting your weight or pacing as these are indications of anxiety and can increase agitation.

5. Position yourself for safety:

    • Never turn your back for any reason.

- Keep a distance from the agitated person to allow you time to react if the person grabs or lunges at you.

- Angle your body and turn slightly sideways in relation to the agitated person. This stance reduces your target size in the event of an attack.

- If you don't have an exit strategy available, position yourself behind a sofa, large chair, table, or desk that can act as a barrier.

6. Practice simple listening. When you are under attack by an aggressor who is trying to vent his frustration by talking, try to listen and pretend to understand the problem instead of ignoring the person and inviting further attack.

7. The tone of your voice is very important when de-escalating a situation. No matter how you feel about the attack, your tone must remain calm so that the attacker gets the impression that you understand and agree with their situation. This will allow you a chance to exit to safety without angering them any further.

If the situation evolves beyond the use of de-escalation and you do have to physically fight back to protect yourself, you must be willing to inflict serious injury to your assailant so that you will have time to escape to safety. If physical defense is needed, you can strike and kick at any of the assailant's body parts, but there are vulnerable target areas to aim for. In order for force to be maximally effective, a strike must be applied to the vulnerable areas of the body. There are also many powerful joint locks and pressure points, but it takes a considerable amount of training and consistent practice to be able to apply these techniques.

The Action Awareness Training *TEN-Second Strike* is easy to remember and can be applied with minimal muscle strength or previous training. It does, however, take a strong attitude on your part, one that clearly demonstrates that you're ready to show the attacker that they picked the wrong woman to mess with.

The TEN-Second Strike: Targeting the Throat, Ears, and Nose

Throat: A chop or any direct strike is effective against the throat because of the vital functions performed by the esophagus, larynx, and thyroid. The simplest way to strike this area is to push your thumb or finger straight into the indentation at the bottom of the throat. This requires little physical strength on your part and can cause a major distraction that can aid in you getting away from an attacker.

Ears: Slightly cup your hands and clap them together as if you're applauding. That's the same motion you want to apply to the ears: simply slap your cupped hands as hard as you can over one ear or both ears. You can also grab an attacker's ears and pull straight down, or you can jam foreign objects into the ear. All of these techniques yield a variety of immobilizing effects as air is forced into the eardrum. Significant or continued blows to the ears can cause a loss of equilibrium.

Nose: Using the palm of your hand, an elbow, or a knee, hit the nose with ample force. This can cause tears to the attacker's eyes and cause bleeding, or confusion and may give you the moment you need to apply another strike or make your escape. These three strikes will take less than ten seconds total to apply, but in reality, when fending off an assailant, most likely you'll need to land repeated strikes before you'll be able to free yourself. *Once you start physically defending yourself, don't stop until you can get away safely.* And remember, it's *smart*—not wimpy—to run if there is somewhere safe to run to. If there is nowhere safe to run, you will have to disable the assailant first and then run.

The TEN-second strike is very effective and can be used by anyone, but it shouldn't take the place of a hands-on self-defense course. Self-defense classes can boost your confidence and provide muscle memory for applying escape techniques. Learning self-defense is also an effective way to acknowledge unhealthy body language and turn your own body language into a naturally powerful presence.

A Note on Weapons

Carrying weapons for self-defense (i.e., firearms, knives, or chemical sprays) may be dangerous unless the person carrying them is trained and proficient in their use. If you choose to carry a weapon, keep in mind that weapons can also be taken from you and used against you.

Exercises to Educate the Body

- Know your body and your abilities. Remember, you don't want two strangers to deal with during an attack, so it's just as important to hone a sense of physical self-awareness as it is to develop emotional awareness. Observe and get to know yourself. How do you respond when you're scared? How does your body language change? How do you respond when you're excited? The better you know yourself, the less likely you are to be caught by surprise and freeze in a situation when your personal safety is in danger and immediate action is required.

• Read up on nutrition. What you put into your body is the fuel that helps keep your mind clear and your body strong. Keep your body healthy from the inside out.

• Study yoga, martial arts, dance, or some form of exercise that strengthens your body-mind connection and encourages a personal relationship with your body.

• Light a candle and take a warm bath. Do something nice for yourself, give your body a chance to de-stress, and encourage calmness and a centered body-mind-spirit connection.

Chapter Three
Empowering the Spirit: Courage

Courage comes from deep within, from a place that is often hidden by distractions and false securities. Courage reveals who you are and who you are really meant to be. You can't always control the situations life throws your way, but you *can* control how you react to them. In Action Awareness Training, courage represents the practice of having a positive attitude, believing in yourself, and having the faith that you can maintain and strengthen your ability to stay safe.

Have you ever thought much about what your thoughts are, where they come from, or what power they have in molding and shaping your life? Have you ever considered the fact that your thoughts are derived from and triggered by pure consciousness? Individual thoughts play a crucial role in determining how each event, condition, and circumstance in our lives unfolds. How much control you have over your thoughts can only be determined by your willingness to become consciously aware of the thoughts you choose to think.

You can never create what you want if your predominant focus is on what you *don't* want. Just like you can't expect an apple tree to produce a peach, you can't expect the seeds of doubt, fear, and limitation to produce a strong foundation of abundance, safety, and awareness. Understanding and learning how to consciously implement the power of your thoughts is a vital component to experiencing and achieving personal safety and well-being.

The well-rehearsed motto "Just say no!" is important and has its time and place, but for now let's instead look at personal safety through the lens of a fresh perspective. How would your life change if your motto was "Just say yes"? Yes, I'll take that new job! Yes, I'm going skydiving! Yes, I feel the need to make a change! Yes, I care enough about myself to eat healthy! Yes, it's a beautiful day! Yes, I love myself! Yes, I'm worth defending!

It sounds easy enough to "just say yes"—until the wavering internal voice pipes up and wants to say "no." That voice has struggled with pre-conditioned damaging beliefs, childhood mishaps, or past relationships gone sour. We can view how easily we can say "yes" to life as a natural test that allows us to access our capacity to believe in ourselves.

Why are self-belief and self-value essential to both our personal safety and our overall happiness? Because we act automatically within the limits of the fundamental beliefs that we develop, especially the beliefs we have about ourselves and our abilities. As a result, we also limit the results we get. If we believe we are likely to fail, our subconscious mind will create actions that support us failing. When the going gets tough (and it usually does at some point in life), we won't go the extra mile we need to succeed if we lack self-belief. Initial failure then supports our belief that we're going to keep failing; at that point, we may give up or only put out a minimal effort. This is obviously a self-devastating tactic should we need to defend ourselves during an attack.

Self-belief is vital! How many things have you not done or missed out on because you lacked self-belief or a sense of self-value? That's when self-doubt and its companion, fear, creep in. Suddenly, you may start to question your abilities and even your self-worth. Your inner voice might start saying things like "Can I really do this?" or "Am I really worth it?" or "I can't risk failure" or "What will other people say and think if I do this?"

"Fear can cause women to restrict their behavior, which can cause a 'fear loop.' That is, the more a person restricts their behavior, the more fearful they become, hence restricting their behavior even more."[8] But the truth of the matter is that nobody can make you feel inferior without your consent.

Self-belief gives you the freedom to make mistakes and cope with obstacles by seeing them for what they are: temporary setbacks and lessons, not the end of the world.[9] Self-belief means descending from the ego and embracing all sides of the self and the situations you have been, or are, involved in. Honoring and acting upon your self-worth, having self-belief, and implementing a positive attitude play crucial roles in the success of your personal safety.

It takes a positive, solution-oriented attitude to create self-belief, and vice versa. Faith is required to maintain this reciprocity and propel it into action so that these two powerful assets can work together to create healthy experiences. This is often easier said than done, because as defined in *Merriam-Webster's Dictionary*, faith is "a firm belief in something for which there is no proof." This requires a trust that is intangible, and doesn't always make sense to the logical mind. In the context of *Stop, Look, and Listen*, faith is less about a specific religious affiliation and more about persistent action, connection, and direction of self.

Self-belief is a set of existing ideas we hold onto; faith looks toward what is to come.

It is not *because* of faith but *through* faith that we continue to move past obstacles, reach our goals, find inner awareness, and manage our survival.

So what does courage *really* represent in Action Awareness Training?

A positive, solution-oriented attitude. Self-belief. Faith (a.k.a. trust).

Your personal safety really *is* in your hands. Even though unforeseen obstacles, challenges, and unpredictable conditions will arise, when we have courage we can cultivate self-belief and trust in the process. It's about embracing yourself and your abilities.

We all possess different gifts, and that's what makes each one of us beautiful, unique, and important to each other's growth and the world we live in. Be proud of who you are!

Exercises to Empower the Spirit

- Give thanks. Whichever religion or belief you're dedicated to, take time in each day to give thanks and connect with a higher source or the love you have for the people in your life.

- Nurture yourself with nature. Get out in nature and pay attention to the sounds and sights around you. Spending time in nature can increase awareness, calm the nerves, and encourage receptivity and openness to new possibilities.

- Try something new! What is it you've always wanted to do? Learn a new profession, paint a picture, play tennis, write a book, skydive, parallel park, build an engine, go back to school, take a dance class . . . the possibilities are endless!

- Practice kindness and compassion by listening without judgment.

- Spend time each day thinking positive thoughts about yourself and where you want to go in life.

- Practice random acts of kindness. (They will come back tenfold!) Send a bouquet of flowers to a friend, help your neighbor carry groceries, pay for the person's toll behind you, or send a "thinking of you" note to a family member.

- Laugh! Spend time with good friends and laugh until your stomach hurts. Try doing this in the morning and approach the day with more spring in your step!

- See a movie or a theatrical performance.

- Get involved in projects, from company volunteer efforts to community programs to school functions. Become a leader and use your voice.

- Change your perspective. Nothing increases courage more than breaking out of your rut and changing your perspective. Do things differently! Take a different route to work, look at the room from the vantage point of a different chair, or switch workspaces with a colleague. This will help take you out of autopilot mode (also known as the "hamster wheel effect") and bring you into the present.

Part Two:
General Safety Tips

Chapter Four

Safety 101

Stop. Look. Listen. This is a 3-second rule that could save your life. Stop. Clear your mind. Look. Check your surrounding environment. Listen. What is your body telling you? What do you feel? Trust your intuition and act on it.

1. Always strive to portray a positive, strong version of yourself. Stand tall and keep your eyes up. Be aware of your surroundings and take mental notes of all the activity around you.

2. Learn basic self-defense moves. If you do have to physically defend yourself, give it your 100 percent effort, and once you've started, don't stop until you are safe.

3. Use your voice. Yelling, screaming, and shouting are some of the most effective ways to diffuse a threatening altercation.

4. Act as though you have a mission, because you do. A mission to protect yourself.

Three Common Approaches Assailants Use to Lure Their Victims

1. The Emergency Lure

When there is an emergency, it requires our immediate attention and a quick response. An attacker can easily catch you off-guard by approaching you with a fake crisis. Someone might say, "Your child has just been in a car accident and I need you to come with me to the hospital!" or "Your house is on fire!" or "There has been a terrible accident at your husband's work and he is asking for you! I came to take you to him."

Assailants count on women to react based on their emotions. Especially in times of crisis, it's vital for our safety to use the *Stop, Look, and Listen* method before making any decisions. Don't go with *anyone* until the emergency is verified. If possible, use your own vehicle.

2. Uniform Fraud

By their very nature, uniforms represent an official identity and often a trusted figure such as that of a policeman or a firefighter. This means that assailants can wear official-looking uniforms or badges to heighten trust levels and quickly disarm our guard. Uniform fraud can be used in conjunction with the emergency lure or by itself. If an electric company service person, a policeman, a Comcast worker, or anyone in uniform shows up at your door and you're not expecting them, don't open the door! Be especially wary if they don't have a company vehicle. Have them slide their card under the door and call the number on it to verify their identity and reason for knocking on your door.

When you're driving and a police officer's flashing lights signal you to pull over, keep driving until you can pull over in a populated area such as a store or restaurant parking lot. Even if you have to drive many miles, a legitimate cop will understand your concern for safety. If you're uncertain about the legitimacy, you can put on your blinker or flashers to acknowledge that you see the officer and show them you are planning to pull over eventually.

3. The Assistance Lure

Women are helpful by nature, and it's a natural response to want to help a person asking for directions or to assist an injured or disabled person or someone who needs help carrying packages. Assailants often use fake disabilities and pretend to need a helping hand in order to lure their victim into their car or home or to an isolated area. On the flip side, an assailant may also offer assistance to you, hoping to get close to you and gain some of your trust and thus mark you an easy victim. Always trust your gut instinct and your intuition. Remember, if it doesn't feel right, it probably isn't right.

Chapter Five

Making Sure You're Safe in Public and at Home

Shopping Smarts

What if you're unknowingly putting yourself in danger just by doing your daily routine? Even shopping in crowded malls or carrying multiple grocery bags and items can make you a target for criminals.

- Never put the straps of a purse around your neck to protect it from theft. The sudden impact on your neck from a potential purse snatcher could cause you serious injury.

- Don't display large amounts of cash—carry only enough money to purchase what you need.

- Avoid using bathrooms that are tucked away in the corner of a store or mall—instead, try to find a bathroom that is by a food court or other well-trafficked area. Always accompany your child into the bathroom.

- Fanny packs can be used to carry valuables while shopping. They leave both hands free, and because they're worn close to the body, they're hard to get off.

- Don't leave valuables in your car. Even items of relatively low value like coins or sunglasses can be enough to tempt a thief.

- Walk around large crowds instead of through the middle. In the middle, it is easy for someone to grab your arm, stick a knife to your side, and order you to continue walking without anyone noticing.

- Carry money in several different locations instead of keeping an entire wad of cash in your wallet. That way, when you make a purchase and get back small amounts of change, it appears to the onlooker that you have spent all your money.

- If you're shopping alone at night—and especially if you're carrying many packages—ask a security guard to walk you to your car.

- Park your car in a well-lit area and make sure to lock your doors.

- After opening the trunk to your car to load your packages, put your keys in your pocket for safekeeping.

- Use shopping carts! If they're available, use a shopping cart to help keep your hands free. They also can be used as a barrier between you and an attacker. If possible, avoid putting your purse in the cart. Keep your purse on you or put your pockets to good use.

- Shop with a friend. It can be lots of fun, plus the buddy system is always a good safety move.

- Approach your vehicle with your keys already in your hand.

*What if...*I notice suspicious activity when leaving a store to go back to my vehicle?

Go back inside the store and ask an employee to accompany you to your car. Alternatively, you may be able to wait a few minutes for the scene to clear. If it's a more intense situation, call the police and wait in the store until they arrive.

*What if...*I am making many purchases and I need to take several trips to put packages in the car?

Keep your packages safe by placing them in the trunk instead of the backseat, where they are visible to everyone. Move your car to another location between visits to the car. By loading packages into your vehicle and then returning to the store, you make yourself a possible target.

*What if...*I am approached by a person with a knife who demands money or my purse?

They want something. The best way to get them to leave is to give them something. Better to have it be something replaceable than yourself.

*What if...*multiple people approach me in a threatening manner when I am walking to my car?

Try to keep each person in your sight without letting them get behind you. Use your car panic alarm, yell, and make a scene to attract attention to you. And remember, it's always best to use the buddy system whenever possible.

Driving Safety

When you're a woman driving alone, car crashes are far from the only risk you face. Carjacking, abduction, and falling prey to a police impersonator all pose additional hazards for women, who are more likely than men to be targeted by sexual predators.

- Always lock your doors when you enter and exit your car. When entering your vehicle, always check the backseat to ensure no one is hiding inside.

- Keep your vehicle's manual in your glove compartment for easy referencing in case of a vehicle breakdown.

- Keep your car well-maintained—a well-maintained car is less likely to break down or give you problems. Keep your car in good mechanical condition and have it serviced regularly.

- Know something about your vehicle. Learn how to change the tires and add oil and coolant. (Or at least have a AAA membership that allows you to call for roadside assistance.)

- Don't pick up hitchhikers. No matter how "nice" they look, you never know what their plan is.

- If you get stranded on the side of the road, open the trunk and hood of your car just enough for people to notice that you need help. If you open either one completely, a vehicle can stop out of your view directly in front of or in back of you and a person can approach you unseen, taking you by surprise.

- Have your keys ready when you approach the car.

You don't want to spend time digging through your purse looking for your keys.

- When driving, stay far enough away from the car in front of you so that you can see where their back tires touch the ground. This should allow enough room for you to maneuver away if need be.

- Always have your cell phone charged in case of emergencies.

- Keep a flashlight, a few dollars in quarters, a map of the city you are in, and twenty dollars in your car. The flashlight can be used as a weapon or a light. The quarters can be used for parking, and the extra cash is for car emergencies such as gas or new windshield wipers.

- Give a family member or friend your travel itinerary and check in with them at prescheduled times.

*What if...*I am headed home and I sense that I'm being followed?

Don't lead the person following you to your home. Instead, drive to the nearest open business, police station, or fire department and go inside.

*What if...*my car breaks down alongside the road and I am waiting for help?

Stay in the car and lock all of the doors. If someone approaches the vehicle, roll down your window just far enough to ask for help. You can also position yourself in the center area of the driver and passenger seats, away from either window.

*What if...*a police officer puts on their lights and expects me to pull over, but I don't know an obvious reason for this and I am on an empty road?

You don't have to pull over as soon as you see flashing lights or hear a siren. If the officer is legit, they won't mind that you drove some miles to the nearest store where it is populated if you were concerned for your safety.

*What if...*I am driving into a car wash?

Please, please always lock your car doors before entering a car wash. What a perfect place to be ambushed or carjacked! Not a single soul would be able to witness the attack.

Safety at Home

Home is where we should feel safe and secure. For this reason, sometimes we let down our guard. Take personal safety precautions and make sure you're not caught by surprise.

- Lights are an effective deterrent. Keep outside lights out of reach and protected so that they can't be broken or tampered with and aim lights downward so that they don't cast shadows.

- Keep your doors and windows closed.

- Trim shrubs and trees away from entrances and windows.

- Never open the door to strangers. Install and use a peephole to see who is at the door.

- If you live in an apartment, avoid being in the laundry room or garage by yourself, especially at night.

- Have deadbolts installed on all doors.

- If you just moved into a new home, change all of your locks immediately. Never tag your house keys with your name and address.

- Don't let service people or solicitors into your home. Get a phone number to call so that you can verify their identity.

- Make sure your answering machine or voicemail message does not indicate that you live alone.

- Do not believe that everyone calling with an exciting promotion or investment opportunity is trustworthy.

- Invest in motion-sensor lights and a good home security system.

- Secure your garage by installing automatic openers or bolt-style locks on each end of the garage doors.

- Install a set of sheer window curtains or window blinds to help prevent people outside from looking in while still allowing light to come in.

- Secure your patio door with a pin-type lock, a key lock, or a steel rod inserted into the door channel.

- Do not leave your garage door open when you are away. An empty garage lets others know you are absent.

- Become familiar with the neighborhood watch program in your community. Neighbors looking out for each other are an effective way to prevent crime. If your community doesn't have a safety watch program, contact your local police. They can help you start one.

- When you're away, set up timers to turn your lights on at night.

- Keep outside lights on at night.

What if...a service person (such as an electric company worker, cable repair person, or even a police officer) unexpectedly knocks on my door and requests my attention for some matter?

Don't forget this number-one rule: *Don't open your door without seeing who is standing on the other side.* Ask for the person to slide their card under the door and call the company to verify the reason for their visit. If it still doesn't feel right, call the police and ask for assistance. Keep your door locked.

What if...I have been away and come home to find something different about my residence, such as the lights on, a gate open, or a door ajar?

DON'T GO IN! Get back in your car and call your local police station. Tell them your concerns, and they will come check it out for you.

What if...I am sleeping and I hear someone breaking into my house?

It's a good idea to have a phone close to your bed. Call 911 or your local emergency number immediately and get out of the house if possible. Use a loud device such as an air horn, siren, car alarm, or any other device that will bring attention to your situation. Another option is to keep a stun gun or a can of pepper spray within arm's reach and shock or spray the intruder if needed.

What if...a stranger bangs on my door screaming that there is an emergency and they need to use my phone?

Don't let strangers into your home no matter what the reason or emergency is. Without opening your door, offer to make an emergency call while they wait outside.

Protect against home burglary by making your home look occupied:

- Use automatic timers on lights when away from home.

- Lower the sounds of your telephone and answering machine so they can't be heard from the outside.

- Place radios on automatic timers and turn up the tunes so they *can* be heard outside.

- If you are gone for more than a day, have a trusted friend pick up your newspaper, mow your lawn, and/or shovel your snow. Put your mail on hold; an overstuffed mailbox is a pretty good sign that you're away.

- Keep a parked car in the driveway if you're taking a flight, riding the train, or traveling in any way without your car. Hiding the car inside the garage lets people know you're not home.

ATM Safety

ATMs are an easy and convenient way to get cash, but they can compromise your safety. Because of the different ways ATMs are installed and the various crime considerations at each location, there is no single formula that can guarantee your security when using an ATM. That's why it is necessary for ATM users to consider the environment around each ATM.

- Protect your ATM card as if it were cash. When you arrive at an ATM, take a look around. If you see anything that makes you uncomfortable or anyone suspicious, don't pull in. Come back later and notify authorities if need be.

- Try to avoid using the ATM by yourself. If possible, avoid using an ATM after dark.

- Protect your PIN. Do not enter the PIN if anyone else can see the screen. Use your body to help shield your PIN from onlookers. If you feel like someone is watching you closely, cancel your transaction and do it at a later time.

- Minimize the time you spend at an ATM by having your card in your hand and resisting the temptation to count the money after it has been dispensed. Stay alert! Every few seconds, look away from your transaction and check your surroundings.

- Don't flash your cash. Avoid counting or displaying large amounts of cash when your transaction is finished.

- As you leave, be on the lookout. If you feel you're being followed, go to a populated area and call the police.

- Don't throw your receipts or any other papers with your name or account numbers on them into a nearby trash can. Keep this info with you.

- If you drive up to an ATM, keep your car doors locked and an eye on your surroundings.

*What if...*an ATM card reader appears unusual or bulky compared to other ATMs?

Check with the bank or credit union or use another ATM. Be wary of "skimming." This is a scam where thieves attach realistic-looking devices to an ATM that are designed to capture your card information and PIN.

*What if...*someone demands my money after I withdraw cash?

Don't argue or fight with the thief. Note the assailant's physical appearance and give them your money. You never know if the assailant has a weapon or how far they will go to get what they want. It's better that they take your money than your life.

Walking Safety

Whether you are walking to work, to school, to the grocery store, or to a friend's house, here are a few simple tips to make sure you get there safely.

- Avoid shortcuts through parks, vacant lots, and other deserted areas.

- Wear reflective gear and also wear light-colored clothing, especially early in the morning or in the evening. Wearing a track suit with reflective stripes, walking shoes with reflective material on the heels, or a reflective belt will make you more visible to oncoming traffic.

- If you are harassed by the occupants of a car, turn around and walk in the other direction. The driver will have to turn around to follow you. Walk into a store or restaurant if they continue to follow you.

- Carry your purse close to you instead of letting it dangle, and avoid carrying extra cash and valuables. Don't wear your purse strap across your neck, as this can become a strangling device.

- Walk in the direction that faces traffic. This is the "rule of the road," and it also keeps you aware of any potentially dangerous vehicles that might be coming toward you.

- Vary your route for safety and enjoyment. This prevents anyone from memorizing your route and knowing the best time to approach you.

- Carry identification and don't wear extra-flashy jewelry.

- Walk with a friend! Walk with someone whenever possible, or walk in areas where other people are nearby. Avoid walking alone, especially if you are depressed, exhausted, intoxicated, or otherwise impaired.

- Don't ever hitchhike or accept rides from people unless you know and trust them.

- Upload a personal safety app such as Sentinel Personal Security SOS, bSafe, Watch Over Me, or My Safetipin. When activated, these safety apps will send your precise GPS location to your preselected contacts and notify them that you are in danger.

*What if...*I feel like I'm being followed on foot?

Avoid isolation. Walk toward well-populated and well-lit areas. If you're downtown, walk into the police station or a store. Call the police if you fear for your safety. Call a taxi or a friend to pick you up. Stand tall and walk fast and with a sense of purpose.

*What if...*occupants in a car harass me while I am walking?

Simply turn around and walk in the other direction. The driver will have to turn around to follow you. Walk into a restaurant or store if they continue to follow you. Obtain a description of any person or vehicle involved, including the car's license plate number. This information can be valuable for law enforcement purposes.

*What if...*someone grabs my arm and threatens me, telling me I have to walk with him quietly or he will use the knife he has thrust against my side?

To avoid being hurt your first instinct may be to comply, and keep silent. But it is suggested to do exactly the opposite. Yell and scream to draw attention to the situation. The attacker wants an easy victim and doesn't want to be seen by witnesses. By causing a scene, you may stop the attacker from further action.

Chapter Six

Safely Using Public Transportation and Ridesharing

Public transportation may not be as enjoyable as commuting in your own personal vehicle, but it eases congestion, reduces emissions, and gives you plenty of quality time to people-watch during your commute instead of getting stressed with road rage. But when you use public transportation or ridesharing, take some precautions to make sure you are safe during your ride and that you reach your destination unharmed.

- When you call Uber or Lyft, be sure you're getting into the right car: see if the license plate, car make and model, and driver's appearance all match the information provided by your app. Uber and Lyft rides can only be requested using their respective apps. Never get into a car where the driver or vehicle doesn't match your app information.

- Ask the Uber or Lyft driver to confirm your name before getting into the car. You can ask, "Who are you here to pick up?"

- Advise a family member, friend, or coworker of your ride and destination. Call them when you leave and when you arrive—that way, if you don't contact them when expected, they will know something is wrong. If you're using ridesharing, share your trip status on the app so that your contact will receive a text notification of your ride and your estimated time of arrival.

- On buses, sit behind the driver or next to the door so that you can quickly exit in case of harassment or emergencies.

- At a bus stop, wait with your back against a wall to avoid being surprised from behind. Stay in a well-lit area while waiting for your ride.

- Be mindful of what you're saying or what information you may be inadvertently giving your fellow commuters when you talk on your cell phone.

- Don't choose the window seat and be blocked in— choose an aisle seat for a quick exit.

- When waiting for public transport to arrive, wait in a coffee shop or other well-lit area where there is safety in numbers.

- Give way to passengers disembarking. This prevents overcrowding and lessens the chance of being pickpocketed.

- Try to travel as lightly as possible to reduce the temptation of possible theft. Also, traveling light means you'll have your hands free if you need to defend yourself.

- Always check a driver's identification, such as the badge or license, before entering a taxi.

- Observe the behavior of those around you. Get a feel for your surroundings and move as soon as possible if you feel uncomfortable.

- When using public transport, dress down so as not to bring any unwanted attention to yourself. Avoid wearing expensive jewelry and clothing.

*What if...*I board public transportation and there are noisy passengers arguing and causing a commotion?

Be aware that this could be a staged diversion to sidetrack you while others try to steal your valuables or harm you. Don't get in the middle of a brawl. If you do, you risk the chance of being the one who's harmed.

*What if...*I am waiting for transportation and there is no wall to lean my back against but there is a bench available?

Remain standing and glance around your surroundings periodically. You're more likely to be able to defend yourself if you're already standing than if you're sitting down. Keep your eyes up and remain alert.

Chapter Seven
Safe Travels

When it comes to traveling, there is no one correct way to ensure safety due to the multiple aspects that are involved— where you'll be traveling, your individual circumstances, and your personal perceptions—but there are precautions you can take.

- For your own safety, try to keep a low profile and blend in with the locals as best you can. Avoid wearing expensive jewelry that might attract unwanted attention.

- It's exciting to travel and see new sights, but use caution while taking photos and selfies. It's easy to get distracted while in awe of the spectacular sights. Keep an eye on your surroundings.

- If possible, bring only one credit card on your trip and leave other credit cards, gas cards, and department store charge cards at home. Social security cards, ID cards, and photographs or other mementos that can't be replaced are also best left at home.

- Always lock away your valuables in your hotel room or cruise ship cabin. Many service personnel have a key to your room or cabin.

- As in your home, if someone knocks on your door, never open it without being certain that the person on the other side is legitimate.

- Don't reveal too much about your travel plans while chatting with other people or on social media. You may be overheard by an opportunistic thief or attacker. Wait until you're back home to share stories and photos of your trip.

- When traveling alone and staying at motels, ask the attendant for all of the room keys and let the attendant know that no one will be joining you later.

- When staying in hotels, request a room on floors two through six. This makes you less prone to theft but also makes you reachable by most fire department ladders. Be aware that ground floors with outside entrances and windows are the most vulnerable to unauthorized entry.

- Keep a copy of your passport in your money belt at all times. Keep the money you expect to use during the day in a wallet, money clip, or small purse in your front pocket instead of the back pocket, where it can more easily be lifted or slashed free with a razor blade. Keep coins separate so you don't have to take out your entire wallet in front of a group of people.

- Make sure all sliding doors and windows are secured and locked. Intruders can climb from balcony to balcony to gain access to a room.

- Socialize in well-populated areas of a cruise ship or hotel. Avoid meeting in an individual's room.

- Ask the hotel concierge for recommendations regarding jogging or walking routes. At night, stay in well-lit and populated areas.

- If you park your car at a hotel and a valet puts a card on your dash, make sure it does not have your room number listed on it. Always keep your room number private.

- Do not leave valuables in your vehicle. Crooks know that rental cars may contain items of value.

- Memorize or write down local emergency numbers so that you will be prepared in any situation.

*What if...*I decide to carry pepper spray while I travel?

Pepper spray can be a useful safety tool, but keep a few things in mind before carrying it. If you have to fumble for it in your purse, you alert the attacker of your intentions and waste time. Do your research and buy a good quality brand – make sure it has a safety pin release so the attacker can't disarm you and use it against you. Purchase two bottles and practice using your pepper spray until you feel confident with how it works. But don't depend fully on any self-defense tool or weapon – trust your body and your wits.

*What if...*I plan to sleep in a train compartment?

Keep the door locked at night while you sleep. Consider booking an individual compartment (although they are much more expensive). Otherwise, you're probably bunking with three other people in that compartment.

*What if...*I have to board a crowded bus or train?

If you are standing, keep your valuables in front of you at all times, not behind your back. If you stop at a rest stop, don't leave valuables on your seat when you get off to stretch your legs. Leave something of low value like a notebook, book, or bandana on your seat to save it.

*What if...*I have to use an elevator?

Always position yourself near the elevator control panel if possible. If attacked, push as many floor buttons as possible. Keep your back to the side wall so that you're not surprised from behind. Observe all passengers when entering an elevator. It's wise to board last and select your floor button last. If someone suspicious enters the elevator, exit as soon as possible.

Chapter Eight
Keeping Your Kids Safe

No parent wants to think about scary what-if scenarios or the possibility that their children might need guidance on how to stay safe in life-threatening situations. But despite our best efforts, no place is 100 percent safe.

- Teach your child to dial 911 for an emergency. Don't refer to it as "nine-eleven"—there is no eleven on a telephone keypad or dial. Always say "9-1-1."

- Post your address by the phone for young children.

- Regularly update the photos and descriptions of your children in your home file. Have sets of fingerprints and footprints made.

- Never leave your children unattended in a public place.

- Choose babysitters with care. Obtain references from family and friends. Once you find a caregiver, drop in unexpectedly to see how your children are doing while the caregiver is there. Ask your children how their experience with the babysitter was. Listen carefully to their responses and watch their body language to see if it matches their verbal response.

- Ask your children "What if . . . ?" questions to see if they understand what to do in emergency situations or if you need to clarify more. Make a game out of it and have fun!

- Teach your children about potential online threats. Learn more about internet safety at www. Netsmartz.org.

- Talk to your kids about online dangers and monitor your children's activity online.

- Encourage your children to tell you if anything they encounter at school or online makes them feel scared, sad, or confused.

- Remind children to use the buddy system. They should take a friend with them if they walk or bike to school.

- Walk the route to and from school with your children and point out safe places to go if they're being followed or need help.

- During family outings, establish an easy-to-remember place where you can meet to check in or to find each other if you should get separated.

- Teach your children that if anyone tries to grab them, they should make a scene by kicking, resisting, and screaming.

- Tour your neighborhood with your children so that they know which neighbors they may visit without you and the neighbors they can run to for help if needed.

What if...there was an emergency and I had to send someone else to pick up my child from school?

Make your best effort to contact the local school office and let them know who will pick up your child. Choose a code word with your child for this type of situation and tell them not to go home with anyone (even if they know the person) unless that adult tells them the designated code word. The code word should be kept simple and easy to remember, such as "apple" or "crayons."

*What if...*I'm concerned that my child may be making dangerous online choices?

Know the warning signs of risky behavior and talk to them openly and honestly about their internet activities. Some common warning signs of online risk-taking behavior include: sudden mood or behavioral changes for the worse; excessively surfing the internet, sending instant messages, or using chat rooms (especially at night); receiving phone calls, presents, or mail from people you don't know; making calls to numbers unknown to you; or making great efforts to circumvent your watchfulness while using their iPad, cell phone, or other devices.

*What if...*I think my child has talked to a predator?

If you have even the slightest feeling that your child may have developed an online romantic relationship, take immediate action. Remind your children of how dangerous it is to have a real-life, face-to-face meeting with someone they met online. Save and print any emails or instant messaging sent by a suspected predator. Check the caller ID on your home phone and on your child's personal devices to see if any unfamiliar phone numbers have called. If they have, contact the police immediately.

Chapter Nine
Avoiding Cyber Predators

The internet has drastically changed the way we interact with the world. It is filled with sources of in-depth knowledge, tools that allow us to express our creativity, and technology that allows us to connect with people all over the world. Yet, along with positive possibilities and connections, the internet also offers its own risks, such as cyber-bullying and online predators.

- According to the *New England Journal of Public Policy*, contact with online predators happens mostly in chat rooms, on social media, or in the chat feature of multiplayer games (*Roblox, Minecraft, Clash of Clans, World of Warcraft*, and so on).

- A firewall and antivirus software can protect your computer, but they won't keep you or your identity safe. Set serious passwords and protect them. Keep passwords private and don't use the same one for all of your security needs.

- When communicating online, use a nickname or a user name that is different from your real name, and always keep personal information such as your home address and phone number confidential.

- Be wary of online sites that request your personal or financial information. No quantity of user settings or "protective" checkboxes can prevent a user from willingly complying with the bad guys. This is what they depend on. Don't say anything online that you wouldn't say in real life.

Chapter Ten

Protecting Yourself from Identity Theft and Scam Artists

To be clear, identity theft *prevention* services don't exist— there's no way to actually prevent your identity from being stolen. What the best identity theft protection services *can* do, though, is ceaselessly monitor your credit and bank accounts and alert you as soon as suspicious behavior arises. The rest is up to you. The best way to avoid getting tricked by scammers, is to know the tricks they use.

- When you are asked to provide personal information, ask how it will be used, why it is needed, who will be sharing it, and how it will be safeguarded.

- Do not be hurried into sending money to claim a prize that is available for only a "few hours."

- Pay attention to your billing cycles. If credit card or utility bills fail to arrive, contact the companies to ensure that the bills have not been illicitly redirected.

- Do not believe that everyone calling with an exciting promotion or investment opportunity is trustworthy.

- Never trust caller ID. Always validate a person's organization by calling them back through an official phone number.

- Shred or burn personal financial information such as receipts, credit card offers, and bank statements.

*What if......*I receive an email, text, or phone call that looks like an important message from my bank or from a well-known business that asks me to type in my password, social security number, credit card number, or login name?

The most common types of scams will target you through fake emails (a technique known as phishing), text messages (smishing) voice calls (vishing), or letters. No matter which technique the scammer uses, you may be pressured to send money, threatened with law enforcement action, told to purchase gift cards and provide codes as a form of payment, asked to cash a check for a stranger or send money via wire transfer, or instructed to make a cash deposit for a sweepstake. The best ways to avoid getting scammed is to not respond. If you're not 100 percent certain of the source of the call, email or text, then hang up the phone, don't click on the link in the email and don't reply to the text message.

*What if...*I think I'm a victim of identity theft?

Report the crime to the police immediately. Cancel your credit cards and have new ones issued. Have your credit cards annotated to reflect the identity theft, and document the steps you take and the expenses you incur to clear your name and reestablish your credit.

Part Three: Safety in Relationships

Chapter Eleven
Safe Dating

When you meet a hot new romantic prospect online or in person, safety precautions are probably not the first thing on your mind. You may be going out on a date with someone you've been chatting with online for months, or someone a mutual acquaintance has set you up with. The truth of the matter, though, is that you're making yourself extremely vulnerable to a stranger.

- Chat on the phone often with your romantic interest. A phone call can reveal much about a person's communication and social skills.

- For a first date, consider going with another couple or with a group of friends if you don't feel right about being alone with your date.

- Suggest meeting for coffee or at a wine bar (but only have one drink so you're 100 percent sober). These are public places, and if you meet there and say goodbye at the door, the entire date takes place in a safe setting.

- Trust your gut feeling! If something doesn't feel right, get out.

- Drive yourself and meet your date so that you aren't stuck if the night doesn't go as planned.

- Meet many times in public places until you feel comfortable with your date before meeting in more intimate locations.

- Start slow! Watch out for someone who seems too good to be true. When you communicate, watch for odd behavior or inconsistencies. If anything makes you feel uncomfortable, walk away for your own safety.

- You don't have to spill all the juicy details about your date, but make sure you tell someone where you're going, with whom, and when you'll be back.

- Clearly communicate your boundaries with your date.

- Drink alcohol sensibly—don't get caught up in a situation you didn't plan on due to your alcohol intake.

- Keep an eye on your drink. Never leave your drink unattended. If you have to use the restroom, finish your drink before leaving the table. Date-rape drugs are easy to drop into a drink, and it's nearly impossible to realize what has happened until it's too late.

- Three of the most common date-rape drugs are Rohypnol (you feel this within 30 minutes of being drugged; you might act as though you are drunk or passed out), GHB (you feel this within 15 minutes of being drugged; it's accompanied by a loss of consciousness, vomiting, and seizures), and Ketamine (this is fast-acting; while you might be aware of what is happening to you, you might be unable to move).

Safe Drinking Tips

- Don't accept drinks from other people.

- Open containers yourself.

- Keep your drink with you at all times.

- Don't share drinks.

- Don't drink from punch bowls or other common, open containers. They may already have drugs in them.

- If someone offers to get you a drink from the bar or at a party, go with the person to order your drink. Watch the drink being poured and carry it yourself.

*What if...*my date fails to provide direct answers to direct questions?

Watch for red flags. If your date provides inconsistent information about their profession, age, marital status, or other personal information, displays anger or intense frustration, or attempts to pressure you, take caution. These are all warning signs that you may be in an unhealthy situation.

*What if...*I feel abnormally intoxicated, dizzy, and/or nauseous during my date?

These are all signs that you may have consumed a date-rape drug. Act immediately. It is possible to lose consciousness quickly, so you should not waste time researching whether their symptoms match those of a date rape drug.

Instead, immediately tell a trusted friend you suspect you may have been drugged. Then call for emergency help and get to a safe place. You can ask a friend for a ride home or go to a public location and tell someone about the drugging. Then, seek emergency medical care.

Chapter Twelve

Recognizing Domestic Abuse Behaviors

It's not always easy to recognize abusive behaviors because domestic abuse is about controlling one's mind and emotions as well as hurting the physical body. Domestic violence and abuse can happen to anyone, yet the problem is often overlooked or denied. Abuse does not discriminate. It affects victims of any age, gender, or economic standing. Because abuse can leave you scared and confused, it can be hard to recognize the signs of it.

You may be in an unhealthy relationship if your partner:

- Calls you names, puts you down, or constantly undermines you and your abilities as a wife, partner, girlfriend, or mother.

- Behaves in an overprotective way or becomes extremely jealous.

- Makes it difficult for you to see your family or friends.

- Prevents you from going where you want to, when you want to, and with whomever you want to.

- Humiliates or embarrasses you in front of other people.

- Denies you access to family assets like bank accounts or credit cards.

- Controls all the finances, forces you to account for what you spend, or takes your money.

- Prevents you from getting a job or going to school.

- Threatens to report you to the authorities for something you didn't do.

- Threatens to kidnap or harm the children.

- Displays weapons as a way of making you afraid or directly threatens you with a weapon.

- Uses anger as a threat to get you to do what they want.

- Destroys personal property or throws things around; grabs, punches, kicks, or chokes you.

- Forces you to have sex or to engage in sexual acts that you don't want to do.

- Denies you access to food, fluids, or sleep.

- Threatens or executes threats to hurt you, your children, your pets, or your family members.

*What if...*my partner's behavior matches only a few of the above points, and my partner shows compassion most of the time?

Your partner does not have to match every single listed behavior for the relationship to be unhealthy. Abusive partners can hurt by using emotional abuse, psychological abuse, economic control, or physical violence. Just one of these factors alone may indicate abuse. Many violent relationships follow a common pattern or cycle. The entire cycle may happen in one day or it may take weeks or months. It is different for every relationship and some relationships don't follow the cycle, but report a constant state of siege with little relief. Below is a brief description of the three phases of the domestic abuse cycle:

1. **Tension.** You may feel like you're walking on eggshells; you may feel fear or guilt. Your partner may intimidate you, make threats, or exhibit unpredictable behavior.

2. **Violence.** This is when there is an explosion of physical violence, violent behavior, or intense emotional/ psychological abuse.

3. **Honeymoon.** This is the phase when your partner turns back into the person you fell in love with. You may even have fun spending time together. The abuser will apologize for or try to make up for their abusive actions. They may even blame you for their abusive actions or deny them.

*What if...*I think I might be involved in an abusive relationship, but I'm not sure?

Talk, talk, talk! Know that you're not alone. If you're uncertain and you don't feel quite right about the relationship you're in, contact your local domestic violence support center. Without any judgment, they will clear up uncertainties and provide tremendous support for your well-being and safety. Look at the questions below to see if you answer "yes" to one or more of them—these are common signs that you're in an abusive or unhealthy relationship.

1. Do you feel afraid of your partner or feel like you have to walk on eggshells around them?

2. Do you believe that you deserve to be mistreated or hurt?

3. Do you avoid talking about certain topics out of fear of angering your partner?

4. Do you feel emotionally alone or helpless?

5. Do you wonder if you're the one going crazy?

*What if...*even through the abuse I see the good in my partner, and I believe with my love and support I can fix the relationship?

It's only natural that you want to help your partner. You may think you're the only one who understands them or that it's your responsibility to fix their problems. But the truth is that by staying and accepting repeated abuse, you're reinforcing and enabling the behavior. The abuse will probably keep happening. Abusers have deep emotional and psychological problems. While change is not impossible, it isn't quick or easy. Change can only happen once your abuser takes full responsibility for their behavior, and seeks professional treatment.

*What if...*my partner threatens to kill me or hurt my family if I leave?

Instilling fear to keep the victim under their control is a common trait of abusers, and it makes it feel very difficult to get help. You can always call 911, and you can make a safety plan before going to a safer environment. Have your bag packed and be ready to walk out the door without looking back. Here are some important items to take when leaving:

1. Identification: driver's license, state ID, passport.

2. Social Security cards: both yours and the children's.

3. Money: checkbooks, ATM cards, cash. If you're married, you can legally take half of the money that's in the savings and checking accounts.

4. Important documents: welfare ID, green cards, medical records, insurance papers.

5. Children's records: including vaccine and school records.

For anonymous, confidential help available 24/7, call the National Domestic Violence Hotline at 1-800-799-7233 (SAFE) or 1-800-787-3224 (TTY).

Chapter Thirteen
Stopping a Stalker

Most stalking is executed by someone known to the victim, such as a current or former partner. Yet some victims are stalked by complete strangers. Stalking can cause a lot of psychological trauma and if it's happening to you, talk to people about your situation. Get help from support groups, friends, and family. You shouldn't have to turn your life upside down and go through this alone.

- Let your local police know about the matter.

- Keep your cell phone charged. Use a personal safety app to notify your family and friends about your concerns and where you currently are, especially when you're traveling. (There are numerous personal safety apps and they are constantly evolving. You can Google "personal safety apps" to find the best fit for your lifestyle and needs.)

- Build your confidence by taking a hands-on self-defense course to learn physical kicks, strikes, and escape techniques.

- Change and strengthen your locks.

- Save any harassing emails, letters, or phone messages in case you need them for legal proof.

- Don't initiate contact! Be aware that any communication from you can easily be misconstrued by the stalker—they will likely think that you are showing interest in them even if your words are expressing the exact opposite.

- Change your schedule and daily routes to make it harder to follow you.

- Contact victim resources in your local area for support and guidance.

*What if...*at times I feel like I'm being watched or followed, but I'm unsure if it's considered stalking?

Research and educate yourself on the wide array of behaviors a stalker may exhibit. For example, does someone always seem to be just around the corner when you are going to work, when you're out with friends, or in your neighborhood? Does someone keep making unwanted phone calls to your home or work? Do you find signs that someone has been in or near your home, your car, or your workplace when you were not there? Has someone tried to get information about you from a third person like a family member, friend, or co-worker? Is someone posting information or spreading rumors about you on the internet, in a public place, or by word of mouth? Are you receiving repeated letters, gifts, cards, social media posts and/or emails even though you told the sender to stop sending them? These are some common ways a stalker may pursue you. If you suspect you're being stalked, but you're still unsure, don't be afraid to speak up. It's better to be safe, than sorry.

*What if...*the person I am dating seems over protective and often wants to know my whereabouts?

Sometime people stalk their boyfriends or girlfriends while they're dating. They check up on them, call or text them all the time and expect instant responses. They may follow them, and keep close track of them even when they haven't made plans to be together. These staking behaviors can be part of an abusive relationship. If this is happening to you or someone you know, talk to someone you trust, or to a victim advocate who will provide support and safety resources.

Conclusion

By using the ABC approach to safety—**A**wareness, **B**ody Confidence, and **C**ourage—you can lessen or possibly eliminate your chance of becoming a victim of crime. If you practice these tips and tools on a daily basis, you will build an assertive mentality and promote prevention. Being able to recognize a threatening situation is half the battle. If confronted with a dangerous situation, having the necessary knowledge to understand your options is a crucial part of your personal safety and well-being.

Although it shouldn't replace a hands-on self-defense course, learning these awareness and prevention tips is an important aspect of staying safe. These tips are also an effective complement to any physical self-defense training. Invest in yourself and take a self-defense class. By practicing physical kicks, strikes, and escape techniques and understanding target areas, you will build knowledge, and knowledge is power. Learning physical defense techniques builds confidence and helps project a non-victim demeanor, lessening your chance of being picked out as a potential victim.

No matter how you choose to continue your personal safety training, may it engage your mind, educate your body, and empower your spirit. You are powerful, brilliant, and brave! You are worth defending, and you have every right to be safe.

References and Bibliography

Notes

1. The National Center for Victims of Crime and Crime Victims Research and Treatment Center, 1992.

2. Stalking Resource Center, The National Center for Victims of Crime, *Stalking Fact Sheet*, http://victimsofcrime.org/ (citing Patricia Traden and Nancy Thoennes, U.S. Dept. of Justice, NCJ 169592, "Stalking in America: Findings from the National Violence Against Women Survey" in 1998).

3. Black, M. C., K. C. Basile, M. J. Breiding, S. G. Smith, M. L. Walters, M. T. Merrick, and M. R. Stevens, *The National Intimate Partner and Sexual Violence Survey* (NISVS): *2010 Summary Report*, retrieved from the Centers for Disease Control and Prevention, National Center for Injury Prevention and Control, 2011.

4. *Uniform Crime Reports*, Federal Bureau of Investigation, 1991.

5. *Violence Against Women, A Majority Staff Report*, Committee on the Judiciary, United States Senate, 102nd Congress, October 1992, p. 3.

6. Seltzer, Ondre, Frequency Energy Medicine™, https://www.ondre.com, 2019.

7. De-escalating Training, June 6, 2011 http://www.sojourneyrecovery.org/staff/training/de-escalation.htm.

8. Hall, R., "It Can Happen to You: Rape Prevention in the Age of Risk Management," *Hypatia*, 19(3) (2004): 1–19.

9. Tyrrell, Mark, "7 Steps to Self-Belief," July 10, 2011, http://www.uncommonhelp.me/articles/self-belief.

Additional References

De Becker, Gavin, *The Gift of Fear* (New York: Dell Publishing, 1997). Liska, Sanchirico, and Reed (1988), as cited in Ferraro, K. F., "Women's fear of Victimization: Shadow of Sexual Assault," Social Forces, 75(2), (1996): 667–690.

Ouellette, Roland, *Management of Aggressive Behavior.* (Power Lake, WI: Performance Dimensions Publishing, 1993).

Stanko (1993), as cited in Rozee, P. D. and M. P. Koss, "Rape: A Century of Resistance," *Psychology of Women Quarterly* 25, (2001): 295–311.

Wolak, Janis, Lindsey Evans, Stephanie Nguyen, and Denise A. Hines, "Online Predators: Myth versus Reality," *New England Journal of Public Policy* 25, no. 1, Article 6 (2013).

Wooden, Kenneth, *Think First and Stay Safe Parent Guide* (Shelburne, VT: Childs Lures Ltd., 2006).

About the Author

Lila Reyna is a self-defense expert and creator of Action Awareness Training, a personal safety and empowerment program. She is the award-winning author of several books, one of which, *Street Sense: Smart Self-Defense for Children,* landed on the USA Best Books list and won the 2016 Parent's Choice Award from *Parents' Resource Guide.* Her 2019 release, *Living Life for You,* is a #1 Amazon Bestseller.

Lila first started training in the martial art of Kuk Sool Won™ over 20 years ago and today holds the rank of 4th Degree Black Belt. She is currently in the testing process for her Master's degree. Lila is also a practitioner of Frequency Energy Medicine™. Through her in-depth knowledge of the martial arts and the healing arts, the foundation of Action Awareness was built.

As a domestic abuse survivor, Lila originally entered the martial arts and healing worlds determined to reclaim her power and learn the skills she needed to protect herself and her children. Throughout her journey, Lila has learned to transform abuse from something that defined her into a force that drives her to make a difference in the lives of women around the globe.

Action Awareness speaking engagements, online classes, and onsite workshops are available. To sign up for her free newsletter or to bring Lila to your area, visit www.lilareyna. com.

Made in the USA
Las Vegas, NV
10 January 2022

41013223R00062